THE ULTIMATE
KETO FOOD
GUIDE

A Beginners Guide To Keto Foods

JAMES ORWELL

Table of Contents

INTRODUCTION

The ketogenic diet is a very low-carb, high-fat diet that shares many similarities with the Atkins and low-carb diets. It involves drastically reducing carbohydrate intake and replacing it with fat. This reduction in carbs puts your body into a metabolic state called ketosis. When this happens, your body becomes incredibly efficient at burning fat for energy. It also turns fat into ketones in the liver, which can supply energy for the brain. Ketogenic diets can cause massive reductions in blood sugar and insulin levels. This, along with the increased ketones, has numerous health benefits. It's no secret that the keto diet helps you lose weight, and quickly. That's one of the main reasons why people are clamoring to try the high-fat, low-carb regime. But the keto diet benefits more than just your waistline. Passing on the bread is also good for your brain and your heart, plus it'll keep you alive for longer.Before we get started,please take the time to download a free copy of my free keto cook. This will allow you put what you learn in this book to use as quickly as possible. The book includes 50+ recipes for all meals. https://dl.bookfunnel.com/4p1lnh7sfm .

Health Benefits of Keto

The ketogenic diet actually originated as a tool for treating neurological diseases such as epilepsy.

Studies have now shown that the diet can have benefits for a wide variety of different health conditions:

Supports weight loss:

 The ketogenic diet may help promote weight loss in several ways, including boosting metabolism and reducing appetite. Ketogenic diets consist of foods that fill a person up and may reduce hunger-stimulating hormones. For these reasons, following a keto diet may reduce appetite and promote weight loss.

In a 2013 meta-analysis of 13 different randomized controlled trials, researchers found that people following ketogenic diets lost 2 pounds (lbs) more than those following low fat diets over 1 year.

Similarly, another review of 11 studies demonstrated that people following a ketogenic diet lost 5 lbs more than those following low-fat diets after 6 months.

Lowers Inflammation:

Inflammation is your body's natural response to an invader it deems harmful. Too much inflammation is bad news. Chronic inflammation — when your body constantly pumps out inflammatory chemicals for months, and even years — is at the root of chronic diseases including certain cancers, heart disease, and diabetes. The keto diet switches off inflammatory pathways, and ketones produce fewer free radicals compared to glucose. Damage from too many free radicals causes inflammation.

Stabilizes Blood Sugar:

Carbs turn into glucose (aka sugar) in the body. Eating too many carbs causes your blood sugar to spike. When you switch from carbs to fat for energy, you stabilize your blood sugar. Keto can be particularly beneficial for diabetics, who have high blood glucose levels. The keto diet may even cure diabetes — many diabetics are able to come off their medication when switching to keto.

Heart disease: When a person follows the ketogenic diet, it is important that they choose healthful foods. Some evidence shows that eating healthful fats, such as avocados instead of less healthful fats, such as pork rinds, can help improve heart health by reducing cholesterol.

A 2017 review of studies of animals and humans on a keto diet showed that some people experienced a significant drop in levels of total cholesterol, low-density lipoprotein (LDL), or bad cholesterol, and triglycerides, and an increase in high-density lipoprotein (HDL), or "good" cholesterol.

High levels of cholesterol can increase the risk of cardiovascular disease. A keto diet's reducing effect on cholesterol may, therefore, reduce a person's risk of heart complications.

However, the review concluded that the positive effects of the diet on heart health depend on diet quality. Therefore, it's important to eat healthful, nutritionally balanced food while following the keto diet.

Cancer:

Researchers have examined the effects of the ketogenic diet in helping prevent or even treat certain cancers.

One study found that the ketogenic diet may be a safe and suitable complementary treatment to use alongside chemotherapy and radiation therapy in people with certain cancers. This is because it would cause more oxidative stress in cancer cells than in normal cells, causing them to die.

A more recent study from 2018 suggests that because the ketogenic diet reduces blood sugar, it could also lower the risk of insulin complications. Insulin is a hormone that controls blood sugar that may have links to some cancers.

Although some research indicates that the ketogenic diet may have some benefit in cancer treatment, studies in this area are limited. Researchers need to carry out more studies to fully understand the potential benefits of the ketogenic diet in cancer prevention and treatment.

Alzheimer's disease:

The keto diet may reduce symptoms of Alzheimer's disease and slow its progression.

Epilepsy:

Research has shown that the ketogenic diet can cause massive reductions in seizures in epileptic children.

Parkinson's disease:

One study found that the diet helped improve symptoms of Parkinson's disease.

Polycystic ovary syndrome:

The ketogenic diet can help reduce insulin levels, which may play a key role in polycystic ovary syndrome.

Brain injuries:

One animal study found that the diet can reduce concussions and aid recovery after brain injury.

Acne:

Acne has several different causes and may have links to diet and blood sugar in some people.

Eating a diet high in processed and refined carbohydrates may alter the balance of gut bacteria and cause blood sugar to rise and fall significantly, both of which can adversely affect skin health.

According to a 2012 study, by decreasing carb intake, a ketogenic diet could reduce acne symptoms in some people.

However, keep in mind that research into many of these areas is far from conclusive.

LIST OF KETOGENIC FOODS

Being on a diet isn't the easiest thing in the world, especially when you don't know what you should eat. We've put together this ketogenic diet food list to help people out there make decisions on what they are eating and shopping for.

Below you can find a quick visual guide to what to eat on a ketogenic diet. Let's go over some of the commonly identifiable items that people use on keto:

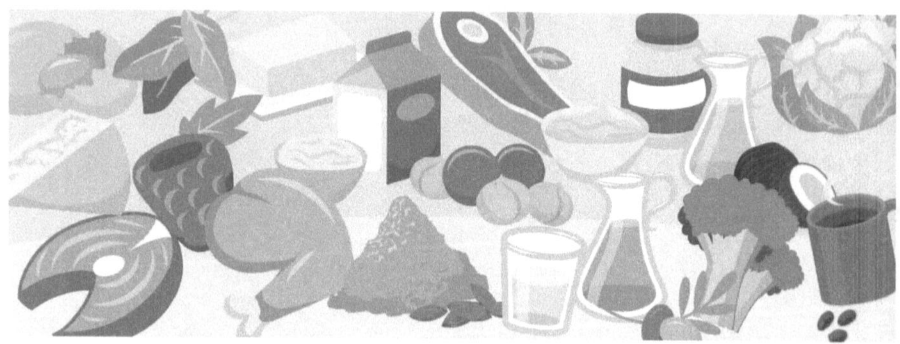

Fats and Oils

Fats will be the majority of your daily calorie intake when you are on a ketogenic diet, so choices should be made with your likes and dislikes in mind. They can be combined in many different ways to add to your meals – sauces, dressings, or just simply topping off a piece of meat with butter.

Fats are vital to our bodies, but they can also be dangerous if you are consuming too much of the wrong types of fats. There are a few different types of fat that are involved in a ketogenic diet. Different foods usually have various combinations of fats, but the unhealthy fats are easy to avoid. Here's a brief overview:

Saturated Fats: Eat these. Some examples of these are butter, ghee, coconut oil, and lard.

Monounsaturated Fats: Eat these. Some examples of these are olive, avocado, and macadamia nut oils.

Polyunsaturated Fats: Know the difference. Naturally occurring polyunsaturated fats in animal protein and fatty fish are great for you, and you should eat these. Processed polyunsaturated fats in "heart healthy" margarine spreads are bad for you.

Trans Fats: Completely avoid. These are processed fats that are chemically altered (hydrogenated) to improve shelf life. Avoid all hydrogenated fats, such as margarine, as they're linked to heart disease.

Saturated and monounsaturated fats such as butter, macadamia nuts, avocado, egg yolks, and coconut oil are more chemically stable and less inflammatory to most people, so they are preferred. Below, you can see some common ways to increase the amounts of fat you eat on a ketogenic diet.

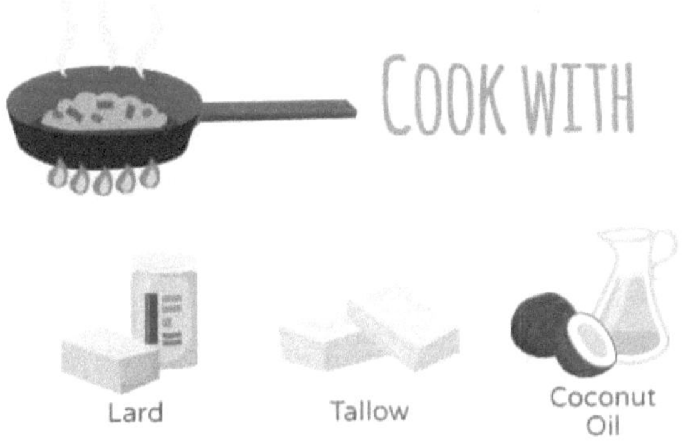

Method#1

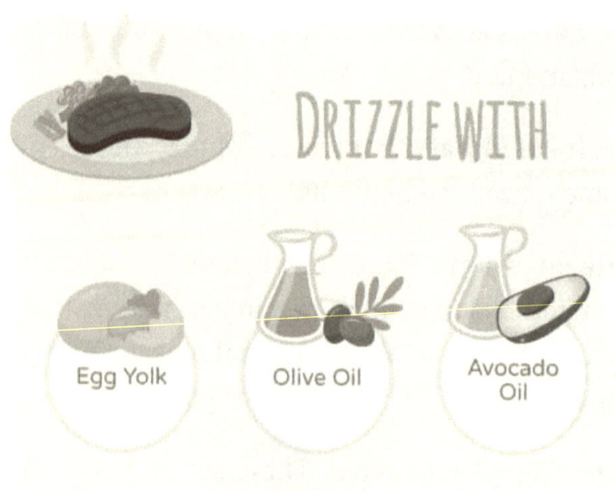

Method#2

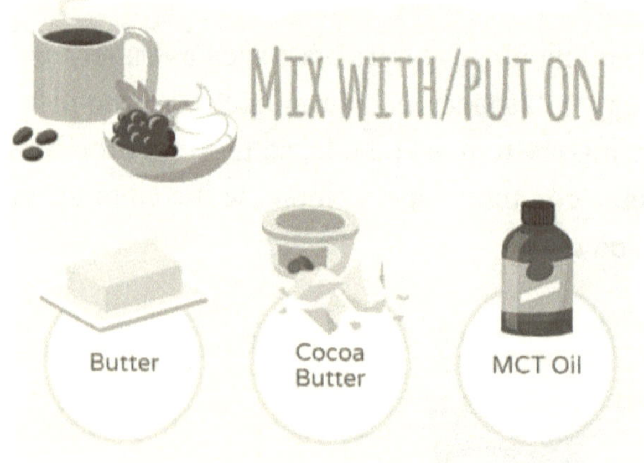

Method#3

You also want to have a balance between your omega 3's and omega 6's, so eating things like wild salmon, tuna, trout, and shellfish can help provide a balanced diet of Omega-3's. If you don't like fish, or just prefer not to eat it, we suggest taking a small fish oil supplement. You can also take krill oil for omega 3's if you are allergic.

Keep an eye on your intake for nut or seed based foods, as they can be quite high in inflammatory omega 6's. These include items like almonds, walnuts, pine nuts, sunflower oil and corn oil. Eating fatty fish and animal meat, keeping snacking to a minimum, and not over-indulging in dessert items that are dense in almond flour is usually enough to keep your omega's at normal ranges.

Essential fatty acids (the omegas) provide core functions to the human body, but they are often times out of balance when on a standard diet. On keto, with a little bit of preparation, your omega fatty acids are easily manageable.

Some ketogenic diet foods that are ideal for fats and oils (organic and grass-fed sources are preferred):

- Fatty Fish

- Animal Fat (non-hydrogenated)

- Lard

- Tallow

- Avocados

- Egg Yolks

- Macadamia/Brazil Nuts

- Butter/Ghee

- Mayonnaise

- Coconut Butter

- Cocoa Butter

- Olive Oil

- Coconut Oil

- Avocado Oil

- Macadamia Oil

- MCT Oil

If you're using vegetable oils (olive, soybean, flax, or safflower) choose the "cold pressed" options if they are available.

If you tend to fry things up, try to go after non-hydrogenated lards, beef tallow, ghee, or coconut oil since they have higher smoke points than other oils. This allows less oxidization of the oils, which means you get more of the essential fatty acids.

Protein

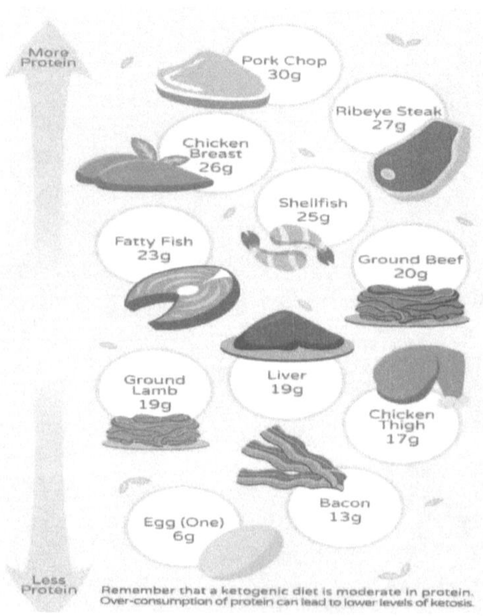

Below, you'll find a visual list of proteins that are commonly consumed on a ketogenic diet. Note that the higher the amount of protein, the less you will want to consume.

Your best bet when it comes to protein is choosing pasture-raised and grass-fed. This will minimize your bacteria and steroid hormone intake. Try to choose the darker meat where possible with poultry, as it is much fattier than white meat. Eating fatty fish is a great way to get omega 3's in as well.

When it comes to red meat, there's not too much to avoid. Cured meats and sausages can sometimes have added sugars and added processed ingredients. If you eat steak, try to choose fattier cuts like ribeye. If you like hamburger meat (ground beef), try to choose fattier ratios like 85/15 or 80/20 in some cases.

One thing you do need to be careful of when dealing with meat is your protein intake. Too much protein on a ketogenic diet can lead to lower levels of ketone production and increased production of glucose. You want to aim for nutritional ketosis, so you must not over-consume on protein.

Try to balance out the protein in your meals with fattier side dishes and sauces. If you choose to eat lean beef, you have to be especially careful with the portioning of protein. Jerky and other beef snacks can add up in protein very fast, so make sure to pair it with something fatty – like cheese!

Note: If you don't eat pork or beef, you can always substitute lamb in its place since it is very fatty. Replace cuts of meat like bacon with similar, leaner items. Add extra fat if needed.

Some examples of how to get your protein in on a ketogenic diet are below:

Fish: Preferably eating anything that is caught wild like catfish, cod, flounder, halibut, mackerel, mahi-mahi, salmon, snapper, trout, and tuna. Fattier fish is better.

Shellfish: Clams, oysters, lobster, crab, scallops, mussels, and squid.

Whole Eggs: Try to get them free-range from the local market if possible. You can prepare them in many different ways like fried, deviled, boiled, poached, and scrambled.

Beef: Ground beef, steak, roasts, and stew meat. Stick with fattier cuts where possible.

Pork: Ground pork, pork loin, pork chops, tenderloin, and ham. Watch out for added sugars and try to stick with fattier cuts.

Poultry: Chicken, duck, quail, pheasant and other wild game.

Offal/Organ: Heart, liver, kidney, and tongue. Offal is one of the best sources of vitamins/nutrients.

Other Meat: Veal, Goat, Lamb, Turkey and other wild game. Stick with fattier cuts where possible.

Bacon and Sausage: Check labels for anything cured in sugar, or if it contains extra fillers. Don't be overly concerned with nitrates.

Nut Butter: Go for natural, unsweetened nuts and try to stick with fattier versions like almond butter and macadamia nut butter. Legumes (peanuts) are high in omega 6's so be careful about over-consumption.

Here's a nutritional list of some of the most commonly consumed proteins on keto and their respective nutritional profile. Keep in mind that you still need to balance your protein intake with fat.

Keto Protein Source	Calories	Fats (g)	Net Carbs (g)	Protein (g)
Ground beef (4 oz., 80/20)	280	23	0	20
Ribeye steak (4 oz.)	330	25	0	27
Bacon (4 oz.)	519	51	0	13
Pork chop (4 oz.)	286	18	0	30
Chicken thigh (4 oz.)	250	20	0	17
Chicken breast (4 oz.)	125	1	0	26
Salmon (4 oz.)	236	15	0	23
Ground lamb (4 oz.)	319	27	0	19
Liver (4 oz.)	135	5	0	19
Egg (1 large)	70	5	0.5	6
Almond butter (2	180	16	4	6

tbsp.)				

15

Vegetables and Fruit

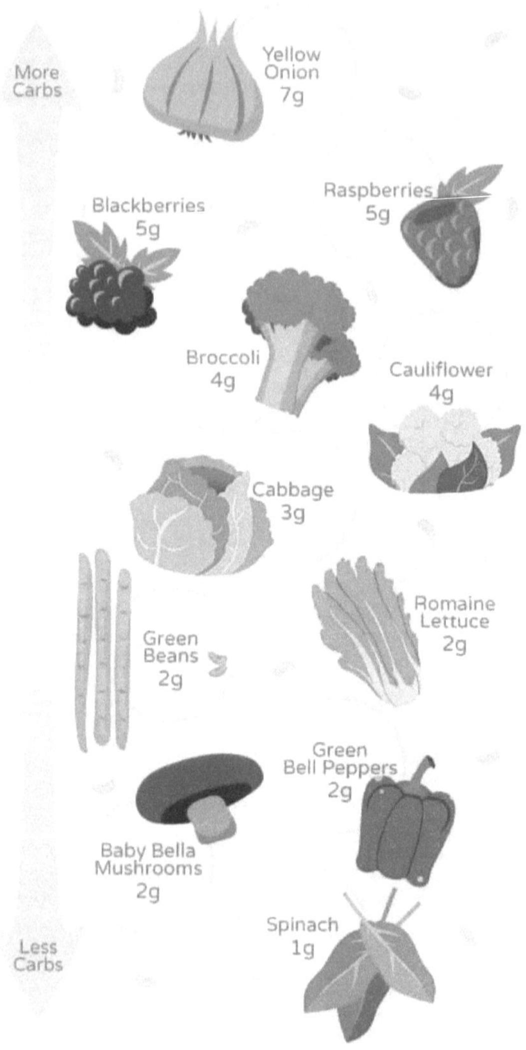

Below, you'll find a visual list of fruit and veggies that are commonly consumed on a ketogenic diet. Note that the higher the amount of carbs, the less you will want to consume.

Vegetables are a paramount part of a healthy keto diet, but sometimes we're stuck with decisions we might regret later. Some vegetables are high in sugar and don't cut it nutritionally – so we need to weed them out.

The best types of vegetables for a ketogenic diet are high in nutrients and low in carbohydrates. These, as most of you can guess, are dark and leafy. Anything that resembles spinach or kale will fall into this category and will be the best thing to include in anything you can.

Try to go after cruciferous vegetables that are grown above ground, leafy, and green. If you can opt for organic as there are fewer pesticide residues, but if you can't then don't worry. Studies show that organic and non-organic vegetables still have the same nutritional qualities. Both frozen and fresh vegetables are good to eat.

Note: Vegetables that grow below ground can still be consumed in moderation – you just have to be careful about the number of carbs that they have. Usually, underground vegetables can be used for flavor (like half an onion for an entire pot of soup) and easily moderated.

In general, there's no fitting rule that works perfectly. Try to choose your vegetables with carbohydrates in mind and portion them based on their carb counts.

Be careful and monitor the vegetables (and their respective carb counts) you add to any of your meals. Especially try to limit your intake of:

- **Higher carb vegetables:** This includes onion, parsnip, garlic, mushrooms, and squash.

- **Nightshades:** This includes tomato, eggplant, and peppers.

- **Berries:** This includes raspberries, blackberries, and blueberries.

- **Citrus:** This includes lemon, lime, and orange juice (or zest) in water and in recipes.

- **Completely avoid** starchy vegetables and large fruits like potatoes and bananas.

Here's a nutritional list of some of the more commonly consumed vegetables on keto. Keep in mind that the weights are the same of everything listed so that it will impact the skew of the carb counts. For example, in a meal you may have 6 oz. of broccoli in the side, but you would not have 6 oz. worth of berries in the morning. You may mix 6 oz. of berries into a pudding with 4 servings.

Keto Veggie/Fruit Source	Calories	Fats (g)	Net Carbs (g)	Protein (g)
Cabbage (6 oz.)	43	0	6	2
Cauliflower (6 oz.)	40	0	6	5
Broccoli (6 oz.)	58	1	7	5
Spinach (6 oz.)	24	0	1	3
Romaine Lettuce (6 oz.)	29	1	2	2
Green Bell Pepper (6 oz.)	33	0	5	1
Baby Bella Mushrooms (6 oz.)	40	0	4	6
Green Beans (6 oz.)	26	0	4	2
Yellow Onion (6 oz.)	68	0	12	2
Blackberries (6 oz.)	73	1	8	2
Raspberries (6 oz.)	88	1	8	2

You may notice that fruits and vegetables that grow underground tend to have higher carb counts, so they must be monitored and limited. To see a full list of low carb vegetables, take a look at the

Vegetable Name	Serving Size	Total Carbs (g)	Fiber (g)	Net Carbs (g)
Broccoli Raab	100g	2.85	2.7	0.15
Watercress	100g	1.29	0.5	0.79
Nopales	100g	3.33	2.2	1.13
Bok Choi	100g	2.18	1	1.18
Celery	100g	2.97	1.6	1.37
Spinach	100g	3.63	2.2	1.43
Mustard Greens	100g	4.67	3.2	1.47
Asparagus	100g	3.88	2.1	1.78

Radish	100g	3.4	1.6	1.8
Avocado	100g	8.64	6.8	1.84
Arugula	100g	3.65	1.6	2.05
Zucchini	100g	3.11	1	2.11
Swiss Chard	100g	3.74	1.6	2.14
Mushrooms	100g	3.26	1	2.26
Kohlrabi	100g	6.2	3.6	2.6
Tomato	100g	3.89	1.2	2.69
Olives	100g	6	3.2	2.8
Eggplant	100g	5.88	3	2.88
Bell Pepper	100g	4.6	1.7	2.9
Cauliflower	100g	4.97	2	2.97
Cabbage (Green)	100g	6.1	3.1	3
Bamboo Shoots	100g	5.2	2.2	3
Cabbage (White)	100g	5.37	2.3	3.07
Cucumber	100g	3.63	0.5	3.13
Jalapeno Pepper	100g	6.5	2.8	3.7
Artichoke Hearts	100g	5.38	1.5	3.88
Broccoli	100g	6.64	2.6	4.04
Bean Sprouts	100g	5.94	1.8	4.14
Fennel	100g	7.3	3.1	4.2
Okra	100g	7.45	3.2	4.25
Green Beans	100g	6.97	2.7	4.27
Turnips	100g	6.43	1.8	4.63
Snow Peas	100g	7.55	2.6	4.95
Brussels Sprouts	100g	8.95	3.8	5.15
Kale	100g	8.75	3.6	5.15
Cabbage (Red)	100g	7.37	2.1	5.27
Pumpkin	100g	7	1	6
Rutabaga	100g	8.62	2.3	6.32
Carrots	100g	9.58	2.8	6.78
Celeriac	100g	9.2	1.8	7.4
Onion	100g	9.34	1.7	7.64
Leek	100g	14.15	1.8	12.35
Ginger	100g	17.77	2	15.77

Dairy Products

Below, you'll find a visual list of dairy that is commonly consumed on a ketogenic diet. Note that the higher the amount of carbs, the less you will want to consume.

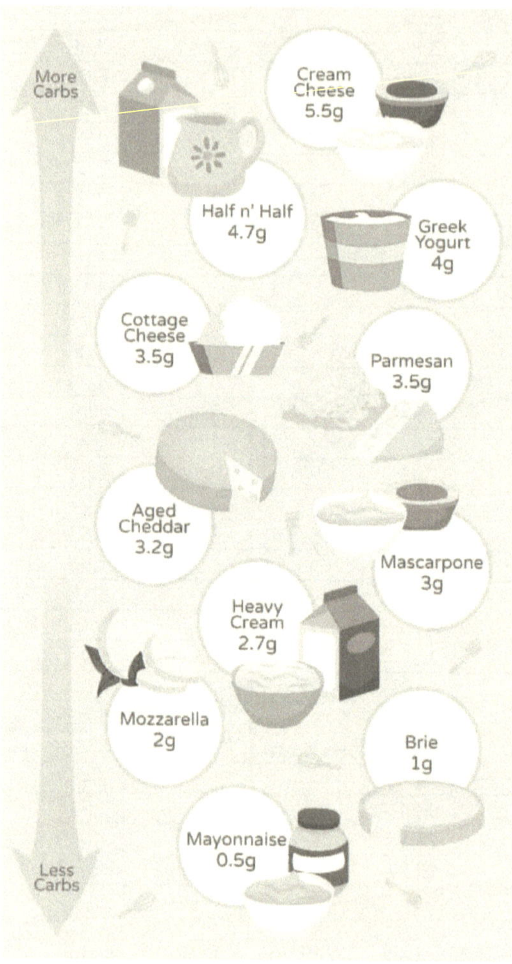

Dairy is commonly consumed in tandem with meals on keto. Try to keep your dairy consumption to a moderate level. Most of your meals should be coming from protein, vegetables, and added fats/cooking oils.

Raw and organic dairy products are preferred here, if available. Highly processed dairy normally has 2-5x the number of carbohydrates as raw/organic dairy so it does add up over time. Make sure to choose full fat products over fat-free or low-fat as they will have significantly more carbs and less "filling" effects.

If you have lactose sensitivities, stick with very hard and long-aged dairy products as they contain much less lactose. Some examples of dairy you can eat on keto are:

- Greek yogurt

- Heavy whipping cream

- Spreadables including cottage cheese, cream cheese, sour cream, mascarpone, creme fraiche, etc.

- Soft Cheese including mozzarella, brie, blue, colby, monterey jack, etc.

- Hard Cheese including aged cheddar, parmesan, feta, swiss, etc.

- Mayonnaise and mayo alternatives that include dairy.

Dairy is a great way to add extra fats into meals by creating sauces or fatty side dishes like creamed spinach, but always remember that it does have protein in it as well. You should always take this into account when pairing dairy with protein-heavy dishes.

Below you'll find a nutritional list of the most commonly consumed dairy items on keto. By far the most common dairy items used are heavy cream (for tea/coffee) and cheese (for added fats in meals).

Note that the nutrition values in the table are based on 1 oz. servings while the visual guide is based on 100g servings (~1/2 cup).

Keto Dairy Source	Calories	Fats (g)	Net Carbs (g)	Protein (g)
Heavy cream (1 oz.)	100	12	0	0
Greek yogurt (1 oz.)	28	1	1	3
Mayonnaise (1 oz.)	180	20	0	0
Half n' half (1 oz.)	40	4	1	1
Cottage cheese (1 oz.)	25	1	1	4
Cream Cheese (1 oz.)	94	9	1	2
Mascarpone (1 oz.)	120	13	0	2
Mozzarella (1 oz.)	70	5	1	5
Brie (1 oz.)	95	8	0	6
Aged Cheddar (1 oz.)	110	9	0	7

| Parmesan (1 oz.) | 110 | 7 | 1 | 10 |

Some people experience slower weight loss when over-consuming cheese. If you notice that you have hit a plateau or slowed down in weight loss, you may want to consider reducing the amount of dairy you eat.

Nuts and Seeds

Below, you'll find a visual list of nuts that are commonly consumed on a ketogenic diet. Note that the higher the amount of carbs, the less you will want to consume.

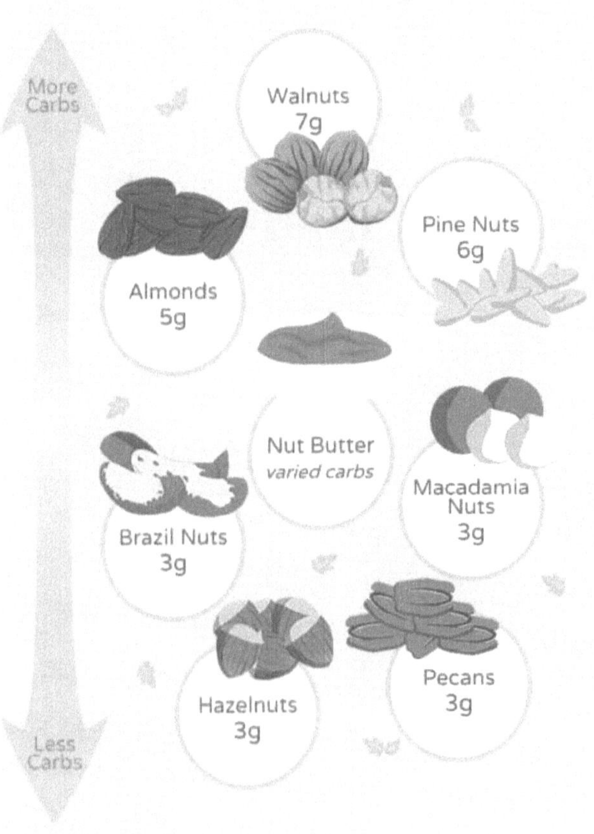

Nuts and seeds are best when they are roasted to remove any anti-nutrients. Try to avoid peanuts if possible, as they are legumes which are not highly permitted in the ketogenic diet food list.

Typically raw nuts can be used to add flavorings or texture to meals. Some people choose to consume them as snacks – which can be rewarding but may work against weight loss goals. Snacking, in general, will raise insulin levels and lead to slower weight loss in the long term.

Nuts can be a great source of fats, but you always have to remember that they do have carbohydrate counts that can add up quickly. It's also particularly important to note that they do contain protein as well. Nut flours especially can add up in protein rather fast – so be wary of the amount you use.

Nuts can also be high in omega 6 fatty acids, so it's good to be careful with the amount you consume. For typical eating, you want to stick with fattier and lower carbohydrate nuts.

Next time you're thinking about opening a new bag of nuts to eat, consider what's better for you on keto from the following:

- **Fatty, low carbohydrate nuts:** Macadamia nuts, brazil nuts, and pecans can be consumed with meals to supplement fat.

- **Fatty, moderate carbohydrate nuts:** Walnuts, almonds, hazelnuts, peanuts, and pine nuts can be used in moderation to supplement for texture or flavor.

- **Higher carbohydrate nuts:** Pistachios and cashews should rarely be eaten or avoided as they're very high in carbohydrates (2 handfuls of cashews is almost a full day's allowance of carbs).

Note: If you have a nut allergy, a common substitution for almond flour is sunflower seed flour. Just keep in mind that this has higher levels of omega 6 fatty acids.

Below you'll see a nutritional list of some examples of the most commonly consumed nuts on keto. Remember that snacking will slow down weight loss:

Keto Nut Source	Calories	Fats (g)	Net Carbs (g)	Protein (g)
Macadamia Nuts (2 oz.)	407	43	3	4
Brazil Nuts (2 oz.)	373	37	3	8
Pecans (2 oz.)	392	41	3	5
Almonds (2 oz.)	328	28	5	12
Hazelnuts (2 oz.)	356	36	3	9

Below, you'll find a visual list of nut and seed flours that are commonly consumed on a ketogenic diet. Note that the higher the amount of carbs, the less you will want to consume.

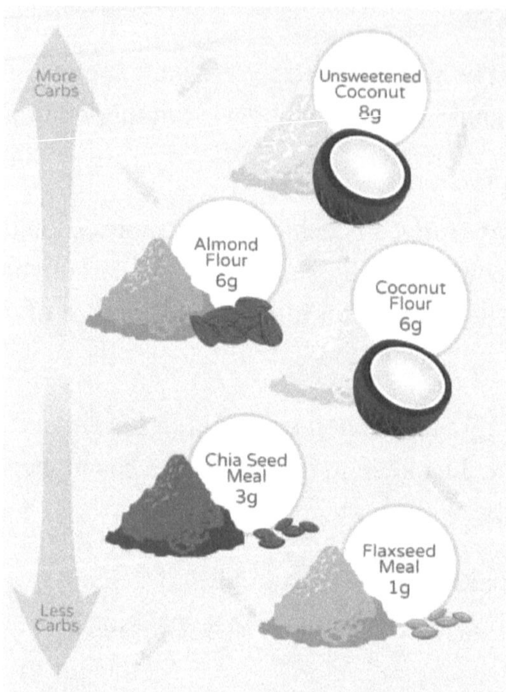

Nut and seed flours are great to substitute for regular flour. Commonly consumed on keto, seeds and nuts are frequently seen in baked recipes and dessert recipes. We often see the use of nuts (in almond flour) and seeds (in flaxseed meal) but should be eaten in moderation.

You can usually use a mix of multiple flours to get a realistic texture in baking recipes. Combining flours and experimenting with your baking can lead to much lower net carb counts in recipes. We think these lemon poppyseed muffins (a mix of almond flour and flaxseed meal) make a great texture when combined with the fats from the heavy cream and butter.

Remember that different flours act in different ways as well. For example, you would only need about half the amount of coconut flour as you would almond flour. Coconut flour is much more absorptive and generally, requires more liquid.

Besides baking, you can also use these flours as a breading when frying foods or even as a pizza base!

You can see a nutritional list of some examples of commonly consumed keto nut/seed items below:

Keto Nut/Seed Baking Source	Calories	Fats (g)	Net Carbs (g)	Protein (g)
Almond Flour (2 oz.)	324	28	6	12
Coconut Flour (2 oz.)	120	4	6	4
Chia Seed Meal (2 oz.)	265	17	3	8
Flaxseed Meal (2 oz.)	224	18	1	8
Unsweetened Coconut (2 oz.)	445	40	8	4

Water and Beverages

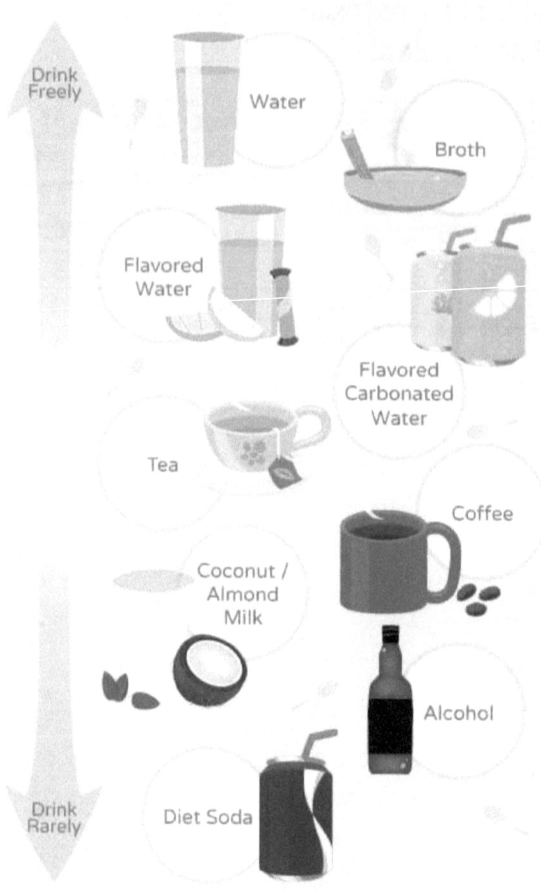

Below, you'll find a visual list of beverages that are commonly consumed on a ketogenic diet. Note that the more restricted they are, the less you will want to consume.

The ketogenic diet has a natural diuretic effect, so dehydration is common for most people starting out. If you're prone to urinary tract infections or bladder pain, you have to be especially prepared.

The eight glasses of water we're recommended to drink? Drink those, and then some more. Considering we're made up of about two-thirds water, hydration plays a substantial role in our everyday life. We recommend that you try to drink as close to a gallon of water a day as possible.

Many people choose ketoproof coffee or tea in the morning to ramp up energy with added fats. While it is a great thing, it's also important to consume flavored beverages in moderation. This is amplified when it comes to caffeine as too much will lead to weight loss stalls; try to limit yourself to a maximum of 2 cups of caffeinated beverages a day.

Note: Many people experience the Keto Flu when transitioning to keto due to dehydration and lack of electrolytes. Make sure that you replenish your electrolytes and drink plenty of fluids. An easy way to do this is by drinking bone broth or sports drinks sweetened with sucralose or stevia.

Some examples of commonly consumed beverages on keto are below:

- **Water:** This will be your staple, go-to source for hydration. You can drink still or sparkling water.

- **Broth:** Loaded with vitamins and nutrients. More importantly, it will kickstart your energy by replenishing your electrolytes.

- **Coffee:** Improves mental focus and has some added weight loss benefits.

- **Tea:** Tea has the same effects as coffee, but many don't enjoy tea. Try to stick with black or green.

- **Coconut/Almond milk:** You can use the unsweetened versions in the carton from the store to replace your favorite dairy beverage.

- **Diet soda:** Try to severely reduce or completely stop drinking this. It can lead to sugar cravings and sometimes insulin spikes in the long run.

- **Flavoring:** The small packets that are flavored with sucralose or stevia are fine. You can alternatively add a squeeze of lemon, lime, or orange to your water bottle.

- **Alcohol:** Choose hard liquor. More beer and wine will be too high carb to consume. Frequent consumption of alcohol will slow weight loss down.

Spices and Cooking

Below, you'll find a visual idea of spices that are commonly consumed on a ketogenic diet. Even small ingredients can add up in carbs; make sure to monitor spices and condiments that you add to your meals.

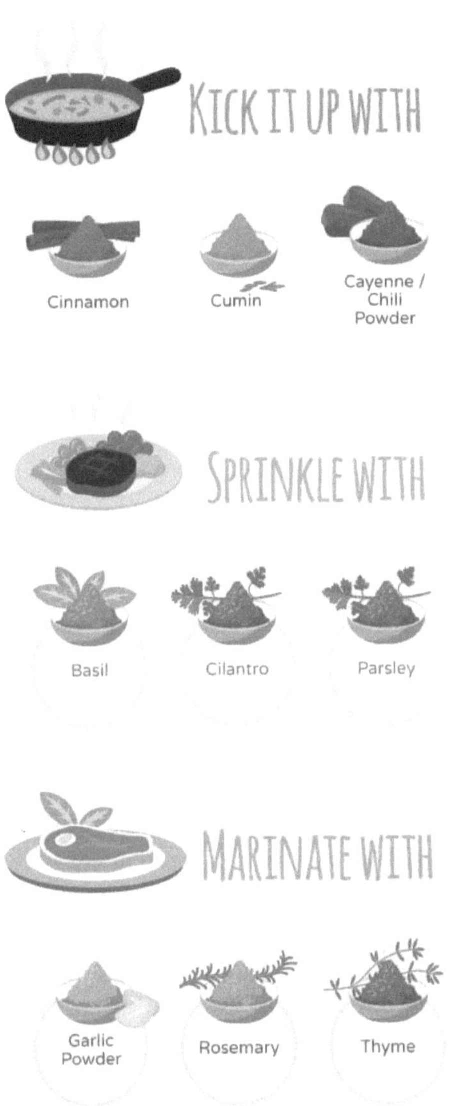

Seasonings and sauces are a tricky part of ketogenic diet foods, but people use them on a regular basis to add flavor to their meals. The easiest way to remain strict here is to avoid processed foods. There are many low carb condiments and products on the market, and there's no way to list them all. A handful of them are great, but the majority use high glycemic index sweeteners – which you want to avoid.

Spices have carbs in them, so make sure you are adding them to your counts. Sea salt is preferred over table salt, as it is usually mixed with powdered dextrose. Most pre-made spice mixes will have sugars added to them, so make sure you read the nutrition label beforehand to make sure you know what's inside. If you have the choice, never include added sugar into your spice blends or food.

Below you'll find some common herbs and spices that people use on a ketogenic diet. Always remember that spices do have carbs in them, so you should make sure to adjust your nutrition based on this.

- Cayenne Pepper

- Chili Powder

- Cinnamon

- Cumin

- Oregano

- Basil

- Cilantro

- Parsley

- Rosemary

- Thyme

Both salt and pepper can be used for seasoning without worrying about the nutritional information.

Typically speaking, the number of carbs in spices is minimal, so you don't have to drive yourself crazy with measuring and recording. When using a lot of spices in a recipe, carbs can add up quickly.

Condiments and Sauces

Below, you'll find a visual idea of condiments that are commonly consumed on a ketogenic diet. Sometimes there is a lot of added sugar in just a teaspoon of sauce; double check nutrition labels to make sure it fits into your macros.

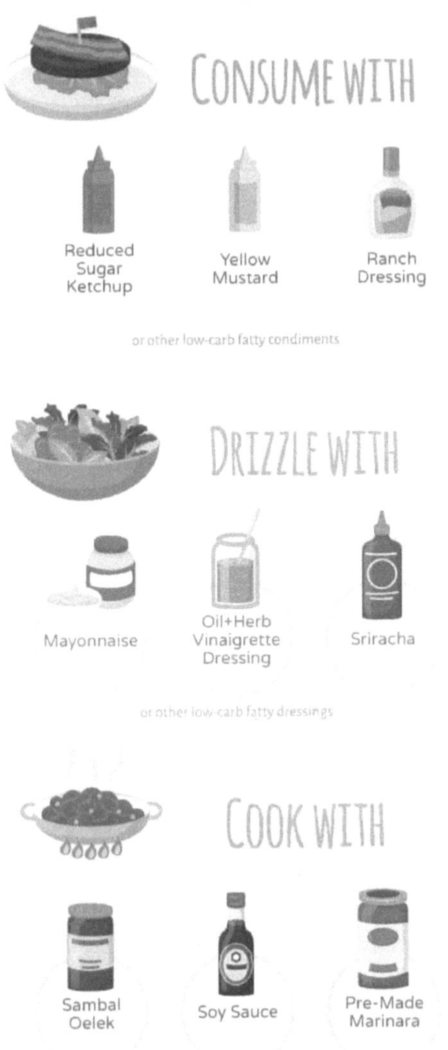

Sauces, gravies, and condiments, on the whole, have a lot of a gray area on keto. Generally, if you want to be strict, you should avoid all pre-made sauces and condiments unless listed below. They can have added sugars or use sweeteners that aren't friendly on the ketogenic diet.

If you choose to make your sauces and gravies, you should consider investing in guar or xanthan gum. It's a thickener that's well known in modern cooking techniques and lends a hand to low carb by thickening otherwise watery sauces. Luckily there are many sauces to choose from that are high fat and low carb. If you're in need of a sauce then consider making a beurre blanc, hollandaise or simply brown butter to top meats with.

Although great in health and theory, you may be like many others and not have the schedule to be able to make everything from scratch. Although it varies from brand to brand (make sure to read the ingredients), standard pre-made condiments for keto include:

- Ketchup (choose low, or no sugar added)

- Mustard

- Hot Sauce

- Mayonnaise (choose cage-free and avocado oil where possible)

- Sauerkraut (choose low, or no sugar added)

- Relish (choose low, or no sugar added)

- Horseradish

- Worcestershire Sauce

- Salad Dressings (choose fattier dressings like ranch, caesar, and unsweetened vinaigrettes)

- Flavored Syrups (choose acceptable sweeteners)

Try to err on the side of caution when it comes to keto condiments that are pre-made. Make your sauces and gravies using thickeners, and try to make your own condiments where applicable. Always double check the nutrition and ingredient list on your food to make sure that it fits in with your dietary requirements.

Sweeteners

Below, you'll find a visual list of sweeteners that are commonly consumed on a ketogenic diet. Note that the less accepted they are, the less you will want to consume.

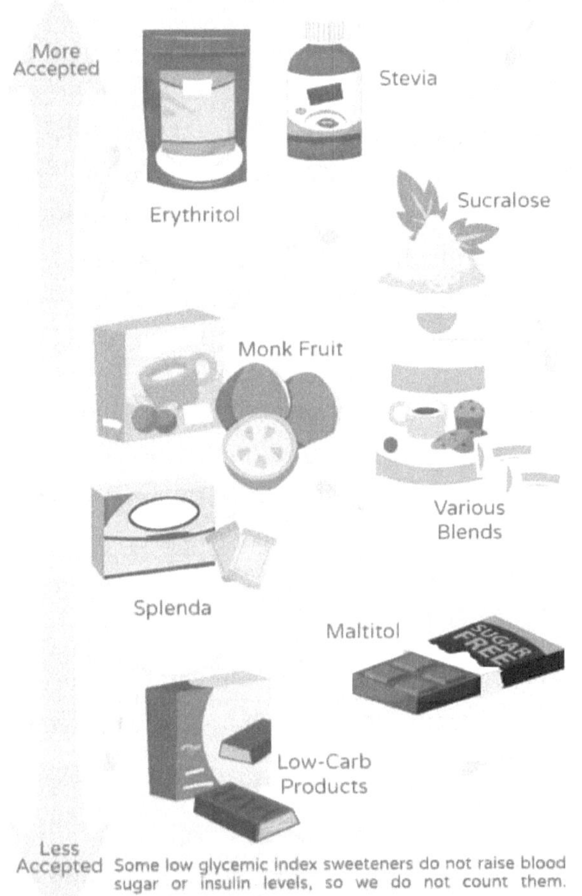

Staying away from anything sweet tasting is the best bet – it will help curb your cravings to a minimal level, which essentially promotes success on the ketogenic diet. If you have to have something sweet, though, there are some options available to choose from.

When searching for sweeteners, try to go after liquid versions as they don't have added binders (such as maltodextrin and dextrose). These are commonly found in blends like Splenda and can add up in carbs very, very quickly. For keto, you want to try to stick with lower glycemic index sweeteners.

Please note that this is just a small list of sweeteners that people use on keto. There are tons of different brands and blends out there – we frequently use a mixture of stevia and erythritol in our dessert recipes. You may find something that suits your tastes better, though, just make sure that it is on the acceptable sweetener list.

Typically you want to stay away from any brands that use filler ingredients like maltodextrin and dextrose, or high glycemic sweeteners like maltitol. Many low-carb products that claim low net carbs usually use these sugar alcohols. Many candies that are "sugar-free" also use these sweeteners. Avoid them where possible. These specific sweeteners respond in our body in a similar way sugar does.

When a sweetener has a low glycemic impact (or a low glycemic index), it has little effect on blood sugar. The higher the glycemic index is, the higher your blood sugar will spike during consumption. Here's our recommended list of 0 GI sweeteners:

- **Stevia.** One of the most common sugar substitutions used on the market today. Incredibly sweet with no glycemic impact. The liquid form is preferred.

- **Sucralose.** A very easy, but very sweet substitution to sugar that has a lot of misinformation around it. Many people confuse this with Splenda, but sucralose is the pure sweetener. Liquid versions are preferred.

- **Erythritol.** This is a great sugar substitution that has 0 glycemic impact. It's special because it passes through our bodies undigested, and is excreted without absorbing the carbs.

- **Monk fruit.** This is a less common sweetener and usually used in combination with others. While somewhat rare, if you can find it, it makes a great balanced sweetener.

- **Various blends.** There are numerous brands on the market that combine these sweeteners in their ratios. Be careful and read the ingredients.

CRAVINGS AND SUGAR ADDICTION

Most of the cravings that we get are caused by sugar. Sugar, at the end of the day, is an industry that's run on addiction. There have been numerous studies showing that sugar stimulates the reward centers of the brain.

When we constantly consume sugar, we release dopamine in our brain – creating an addiction and an increased tolerance. Over time you will have to eat larger and larger amounts of sugar to continue the dopamine secretion. Once our body is dependent on a chemical reaction in the brain, we can find that we're craving things even when we're not hungry.

When trying to shift from a high carb diet to a ketogenic diet, cravings can definitely get strong. It's always best to try to clean house before you start so that you don't have food around you that can lead to cravings. We recommend that when switching to keto, you restrict using sweeteners completely for the first 30 days. It normally leads to breaking sugar addiction and ultimately not having cravings.

Besides sugar, sometimes our bodies crave food because of lack of nutrients. The craving usually goes away if you fulfill your nutrient intake in a different way. Below you'll see a few ways to get rid of pesky cravings that hit.

What you are craving	What you need	What to eat
Chocolate	Magnesium	Nuts,Seeds
Sugary Foods	Chromium, Carbon, Phosphorus, Sulphur, Tryptophan	Broccoli, Cheese, Chicken
Breads, Pasta,	Nitrogen	High Protein Meat

Carbs		
Oily/Fatty Foods	Calcium	Cheese, Broccoli, Spinach
Salty Foods	Chloride, Silicon	Fish, Nuts, Seeds

FOODS TO AVOID

By now, you should have a pretty good idea of what to eat on a ketogenic diet. Make sure that you read and re-read through the list of acceptable foods to build a mental image around what type of meals you will want to eat.

If you're still unsure about any products or food items that might not be keto friendly, don't worry too much. Below, you'll find a list of things that you should always be on the look out for.

- **Sugar.** It's typically found in soda, juice, sports drinks, candy, chocolate, and ice cream. Anything that's processed and sweet you can think of most likely contains sugar. Avoid sugar at all costs.

- **Grains.** Any wheat products (bread or buns), pasta, cereal, cakes, pastries, rice, corn, and beer should be avoided. This includes whole grains like wheat, rye, barley, buckwheat, and quinoa.

- **Starch.** Avoid vegetables (like potatoes and yams) and other things like oats, muesli, etc. Some root vegetables are okay in moderation – be sure to read the section on vegetables.

- **Trans Fats.** Margarine or any other spreadable replacement butter should be avoided as they contain hydrogenated fats (bad for us).

- **Fruit.** Avoid any large fruits (apples, oranges, bananas) as they're extremely high in sugar. Some berries can be consumed in moderation – be sure to read the section on fruits.

- **Low-fat foods.** These tend to be much higher in carbs and sugar than full-fat versions. Make sure you read the package to make sure a mistake isn't made.

www.ingramcontent.com/pod-product-compliance
Lightning Source LLC
Chambersburg PA
CBHW051134250726
48655CB00007B/3050